Published By Adam Gilbin

@ Eddie Keys

Low Carb Diets: The Easiest Way to Lose Weight
and Easy Low-carb Recipes for a Healthy and
Sustainable Diet

All Right RESERVED

ISBN 978-1-990666-69-8

I0554705

TABLE OF CONTENTS

Phony Macaroni And Cheese

Ingredients:

- Salt and pepper to taste

- ¼ cup of heavy cream

- 2 eggs

- 2 cups of cheddar cheese

- 1 1b tofu, firm-well drained

- Cayenee-to taste

- Dry mustard to taste

- Nutmeg to taste

- Onion and garlic to taste

- Use good tofu for this recipes, also use extra sharp cheese to liven up the flavor of tofu

Directions:

1. Tofu should be well drained, ensure all extra moisture is squeezed out, slice it into small pieces.
2. With the use of a separate bowls, cheese, egg and cream should be mixed well.
3. Tofu pieces should be stirred into mixture and then get seasoning added as you wish.
4. This mixture should then be transferred into a greased pie plate and should be baked at 375 degrees for about 45 minutes till it becomes golden brown.

Bacon Cheeseburger

Ingredients:

- 4 oz. of mozzarella cheese

- 4 oz. of cheddar cheese

- 1 egg

- 1 1b ground beef

- Garlic powder, salt and pepper

- 4 slices of bacon

Directions:

1. Oven should be preheated to about 350 degrees
2. Bacon should be precooked in a microwave
3. After cooking, bacon should be crumbled and set aside as toppings
4. Using a large skillet, brown ground beef and get the remaining fat drained

5. It should then be mixed in cheddar, egg, garlic powder, salt and pepper to taste

6. It will then be transferred to a glass casserole dish and will be topped with mozzarella

7. Baking will be done for about 30 to 35 minutes

8. It will then be topped with bacon crumbles

Stir Fry Eggs & Vegetables

Ingredients:

- Cayenne powder, to taste

- Salt, to taste

- Pepper, to taste

- 2 tablespoon Coconut oil

- 4 eggs

- ½ cup spinach, finely chopped

- ½ cup Frozen Vegetable Mix (green beans, cauliflower, carrots, broccoli), thawed

Directions:

1. Pour the coconut oil into a frying pan and heat over a medium high flame until lightly smoking.

2. Add the thawed mixed vegetables into the pan and heat for a few minutes.

3. Pour in the eggs and lightly scramble using a wooden spoon.

4. Add the salt, pepper and cayenne into the pan and mix well.

5. Add the chopped spinach to the pan and stir fry until cooked through.

6. Serve hot.

7. Enjoy!

Sausage & Egg Breakfast Bites

Ingredients:

- 5 eggs

- 1 cup uncooked sausage, crumbled

- Parsley, thyme, oregano or any other fresh herb to taste.

- 1 tablespoon olive oil + some for greasing

- 1/4 cup dark leafy greens, such as Swiss chard, kale, spinach, beet greens

Directions:

1. Crank up your oven to 375 degrees F and allow the oven to preheat.

2. Remove the stems from the greens and cut into strips.

3. Pour the olive oil into a pan and add the greens to the pan and toss well for a few minutes.

4. Add the crumbled sausage into the pan and heat until the sausage is cooked through.

5. Take the pan off the flame.

6. Whisk the eggs with a wire whisk and add the cooked sausage and greens to the eggs.

7. Grease an 8 x 8 inch pan with some oil.

8. Pour the eggs; veggie and sausage mix into the pan.

9. Pop the pan into the preheated oven and bake for about 25 to 30 minutes or until the egg is set.

10. Remove the pan from the oven and cool for a few minutes. Cut the prepared baked eggs into wedges and serve immediately.

11. Enjoy!

Guilt Free, Gluten Free, Low Carb, High Protein Pizza

Ingredients:

For the pizza crust

- lower in carbs utilize 1 cup cooked and squashed cauliflower

- Salt pepper to your preference

- 3 medium zucchini, ground per cup

- 1 egg, and 4 egg whites

- 1 cup White Beans or Black Eyed Peas (pounded/mixed to make a smooth consistency) to make this even

For the pizza toppings:

- 2 cup spinach

- 1 cup mushrooms

- ½ red pepper

- 6 oz. chicken cooked breast

- 45g goat cheddar (optional)

- ½ cup Tomato Sauce (search for low carb/low sugar)

- 1 tsp. dry oregano

- 1 tsp. garlic powder

- ½ onion

Directions:
1. Preheat stove to 375F.
2. Spray a pizza skillet with cooking shower (I simply utilize a couple of pie plate and make individual pizzas).
3. Mix very much ground zucchini, beans (or cauliflower) with egg and egg whites (or mix together), salt and pepper
4. Place zucchini/bean blend on the pizza container fanning out to the edges of the pan.
5. Bake at 375F for 30 minutes.

6. Make pizza sauce by consolidating pureed tomatoes with oregano and garlic powder (add anything more you like). Spread pizza sauce on to some extent cooked "outside" to inside about ½ inch of the edge.

7. Dice veggies and chicken and blend in with goat cheddar. Add fixings to the pizza.

8. Bake for an additional 30 minutes or until cheddar is softened and veggies are delicate and cooked to your liking.

9. You can truly explore different avenues regarding this formula by adding a variety of garnishes and flavors. Get motivations from customary pizza fixings and attempt BBQ pizza, meat sweethearts etc.

10. If you use pie plate, you can just cover with foil and store in the cooler which makes it extremely helpful to get one and go.

Turkey Meatballs

Ingredients:

- 2 tbsp. of stew garlic sauce or hot sauce

- 2 tsp. of fish sauce

- 1 lb. of ground turkey

- 3 tsp. of cornstarch

- 2 tsp. of cilantro

- 1 lemon 1 tbsp. of ground lemon peel

- 2 green onions

- 2 garlic cloves

- 1 egg

Directions:

1. Mix lemon grind, onion, garlic
2. Whisk egg, stew sauce and fish sauce and add to lemon/onion/garlic mix
3. Add turkey blend in

4. Add cornstarch and cilantro
5. Make meatballs and cook for 20-30min 400 degree

Peppercorn Chicken Broth

Ingredients:

- Peppercorns 1 tbs

- Chicken Broth 2 cups

Directions:

1. Place both Ingredients: in a pot and turn it to high heat until it starts to boil.

2. Lower the heat down to a simmer and let it cook for 10 minutes.

3. Take the pot off the heat and then strain out the peppercorns. Allow this to cool and then sip when needed.

Non-Alcoholic Lime-Mint Mojito

Ingredients:

- Natural sweetener ½ cup

- Water 2 cups

- Lime juice 1 oz

- Fresh mint leaves ½ cup

Directions:

1. Place the water and sweetener in a pot and allow it to boil for around five minutes, or until it has thickened into a syrup.

2. Place the mint leaves in a glass jar and pour in the syrup.

3. Cover the jar and allow it to steep for at least 10 minutes. You can use this now, or you can save it for later.

4. Place ice in a glass and pour in a tablespoon of the syrup and a half cup of cold water.

5. Add in the lime juice and mix everything together.

6. You can adjust the syrup and lime juice to your preference.

Zucchini Pancakes

Ingredients:

- 1 pinch ground nutmeg

- 1 pinch onion powder

- Ground black pepper to taste

- 1 tablespoon butter

- 1 teaspoon olive oil, or as needed

- 1 pound zucchini, grated

- Salt to taste

- ¼ cup freshly grated parmesan cheese

- 2 eggs

- 2 green onions, chopped

- 3 cloves garlic, chopped

- 4 leaves basil, chopped

Directions:

1. Squeeze grated zucchini in paper towels to release as much water as possible.

2. Spread zucchini on fresh paper towels and sprinkle with salt; let sit for 30 minutes to release additional water; squeeze again.

3. Mix Parmesan cheese, eggs, green onions, garlic, basil, nutmeg, onion powder, and black pepper in a bowl; add zucchini. Stir to combine.

4. Heat butter and olive oil in a frying pan over medium heat.

5. Form golf ball-sized zucchini patties and place in hot frying pan. Fry until browned, 2 to 3 minutes per side.

Cheesecake

Ingredients:

For the Crust:

- 3 tablespoons powdered erythritol sweetener

- 1 teaspoon vanilla extract

- 2 cups blanched almond flour

- ⅓ cup butter, melted

For the Filling:

- 1 tablespoon lemon juice

- 1 teaspoon vanilla extract

- ¼ teaspoon lemon zest

- 4 (8 ounce) packages cream cheese, softened

- 1 ¼ cups powdered erythritol sweetener

- 3 large eggs

Directions:

1. Preheat the oven to 350 degrees F (175 degrees C).

2. Grease a 9-inch springform pan. Line the bottom with parchment paper.

3. Wrap the bottom and sides of the pan with aluminum foil if worried about leakage.

4. Stir almond flour, butter, erythritol, and vanilla extract together in a small bowl until well combined; the mixture will be crumbly.

5. Press into the prepared pan bottom.

6. Bake on the center rack until in the preheated oven until just golden, 10 to 12 minutes. Allow to cool for 10 minutes.

7. Meanwhile, beat cream cheese and powdered sweetener together using an electric stand or hand mixer at low speed until fluffy.

8. Beat in eggs, 1 at a time. Add lemon juice, vanilla extract, and lemon zest. Beat until well combined.

9. Bake on the center rack in the preheated oven until center is almost set and slightly jiggly in the center, 45 to 55 minutes.

10. Remove from the oven and let cool in the pan. Keep in the pan, cover, and refrigerate to fully set, at least 4 hours, to overnight.

11. Run a knife gently around the sides to remove, unclamp, and carefully remove the pan; it should come right off.

Avocado And Ham

Ingredients:

- 1/2 cup minced ham
- 4 Tbsp diced tomato
- 1 avocado, cored, stripped and sliced
- Paprika
- 4 Tbsp harsh cream
- 4 eggs
- Salt

Directions:

1. Season the sharp cream with salt and paprika. Beat the eggs with a fork.
2. Grease nonstick skillet and spot over medium-high hotness.
3. To really look at availability, add a drop of water and watch on the off chance that it sizzles.

4. Empty the eggs into the skillet and slant to spread uniformly across the bottom.

5. Let the edges set then, at that point, lift it and slant to cook the runny piece of the egg. Set heat on the least conceivable setting.

6. Add the tomato and ham. Set a cover on the skillet and set the hotness on low.

7. Cook for 1 moment or until top is set. Put the cut avocado on top and overlay the omelet.

8. Spoon sharp cream on top before serving.

Country Scrambled

Ingredients:

- 1/8 cup diced green pepper

- 2 eggs, beaten

- 1/2 Tbsp butter

- 1/8 cup diced cooked ham

- Salt

- Pepper

Directions:

1. Place a skillet over medium hotness and soften the margarine.
2. Saute the ham, green pepper, and onion until onion becomes soft.
3. Add the beaten eggs and scramble until set.
4. Season with salt and pepper, and serve.

The Simple Low Carb, Keto Waffle

Ingredients:

- 2 oz. of cream cheese

- 2 tbsp. of Mayo

- 2 large eggs

- 2 tbsp. of your ketogenic toppings (sugar-free syrup or butter preferred).

Directions:

1. Get your blender or a magic bullet, and inside, toss the eggs alongside the cream cheese.
2. You don't have to bring the Ingredients: to room temperature.
3. Blend the cheese and egg mixture until you can achieve a thin and bubbly batter.
4. Allow the dough to rest for some minutes (about 5 minutes), and while this is going on, bring out your Waffle maker, and preheat it for about 5 minutes.

5. When the Waffle maker is hot, and once the waffle maker has been heated up, simply pour the batch inside it (the size of the batch you pour should depend on the extent of the waffle maker).

6. If you don't have a huge Cuisine waffle maker, you need to adjust the pouring of the waffle batch, and sometimes you may have to make two batches of waffle (if you are doing something for your friends and family).

7. Close the waffle maker lid, and wait for a few moments until you no longer see any steam coming out.

8. Put on the waffle plate and then top up if necessary.

9. Serve the waffles immediately.

10. You need to take note of the fact that these waffles may not come out as crispy like some other waffles, however, they will get out better and more crispy if you make use of a

toaster oven, this only means, you can take advantage of the waffle maker, and then toast them in the toaster oven anytime you want.

Gluten-Free Low-Carb Cinnamon Faux-St Crunch Cereal

Ingredients:

- 2 tbsp. of ground cinnamon
- 1 tbsp. of coconut oil.
- ½ a cup of apple juice
- ½ a cup of flax seed (milled)
- ½ a cup of hemp seeds (hulled)

Directions:

1. Get a blender, magic bullet, or food processor, then combine all the dry ingredient inside, then add the coconut oil with apple juice and blend perfectly well until it has achieved a smooth consistency.

2. Put a parchment paper on cookie sheet and spread the batter on top press them down and make then thin in sizes. Bake the batter in

an oven that has been pre-heated to around 350 degrees F, and for about 15 minutes.

3. Reduce the heat to around 250 degrees F, and then bake further for about 10 minutes.

4. With the aid of a knife or cutter for pizza, gently remove the baked crunch cereal from the oven and cut them into squares.

5. Turn on the oven back and put the crunch cereal back and bake further for an hour until they become crispy and break easily (if they remain soft after cooking for about an hour, only return to the oven and cook until it is completely crispy and dried.

6. You may want to serve them with coconut milk or unsweetened almond.

Zucchini Pancakes

Ingredients:

- 2 eggs slightly beaten
- 1/4 cup Carbquik
- 1/2 teaspoon baking powder
- 1 cup zucchini grated
- 1 tablespoon onion minced
- Dash onion powder, garlic powder, salt and pepper

Directions:

1. Heat a greased skillet. Mix all Ingredients: together until well combined.
2. Drop by large spoonfuls onto the skillet.
3. When pancake is brown on one side, flip over and cook until brown on other side.

Avocado Omelet

Ingredients:

- 1 teaspoon lemon juice

- ¼ avocado, diced

- 2 tablespoons plain whole-milk Greek yogurt

- 2 large eggs

- 1 teaspoon low-fat milk

- ⅛ teaspoon salt, divided

- 2 teaspoons extra-virgin olive oil, divided

- ½ cup arugula

Directions:

1. Beat eggs with milk and a pinch of salt in a small bowl.

2. Heat a teaspoon of oil in a small nonstick skillet over medium heat.

3. Add the egg mixture and cook until the bottom is set and the center is still a bit runny, 1 to 2 minutes.
4. Flip the omelet over and cook until set, about 30 seconds more. Transfer to a plate.
5. Toss arugula with the remaining 1 teaspoon oil lemon juice in a small bowl.
6. Top the omelet with avocado, yogurt, the arugula and the remaining pinch of salt.

Cinnamon Butter Fat Bombs

Ingredients:

- 1 tablespoon of Cinnamon

- 1 pound of Grass-Fed Salted Butter

- 1 1/2 teaspoons of Vanilla Extract

- 1/4 cup of Honey

Directions:

1. Allow your margarine to soften.

2. Add your spread, cinnamon, honey, and vanilla concentrate to your food processor.

3. Process for a few minutes to blend your fixings and accomplish a somewhat whipped taste.

4. Stop your food processor as important to scratch down the bowl and reincorporate Ingredients:.

5. Spoon your margarine blend into silicone molds.

6. Then again, you can line a cutting board or level surface with your material paper and afterward spoon spots of your margarine blend onto your material paper.

7. Freeze for a little while, then, at that point, eliminate from your material paper or shape and store in a holder in your freezer.

Protein Sandwich

Ingredients:

- 10g iceberg lettuce

- 1 egg size m

- Salt and pepper

- 75g protein bread

- 50g of grainy cream cheese

- 20g radishes

- 15g rocket

Directions:

1. First fry the egg in the pan.

2. Season a little with salt and pepper while frying. Ideally, shape the egg so that it is optimally distributed over the whole bun.

3. Then remove the lettuce leaf and wash it thoroughly with the radishes and rocket.

4. Then cut everything into bite-sized pieces.

5. As a last step, brush the bread generously with the grainy cream cheese.

6. Now cover: first place the lettuce and rocket, then the egg.

7. Garnish with the radishes and, for those who like it spicy, with salt, pepper or other spices.

Av-Qui Buddha Bowl

Ingredients:

- 30g lamb's lettuce

- 30g paprika

- 15g quinoa (colored)

- 1 lime

- 1 egg

- 50g avocado

- 40g gouda (young)

- 30g carrots

- 30g cucumber

- Sea salt and pepper

Directions:

1. First bring a saucepan with water to the boil and then boil the egg for about 8-10 minutes.

2. Wash the quinoa thoroughly in a very fine sieve under running water.

3. After it is completely clean, place in a saucepan covered with water and simmer for 5-10 minutes.

4. Then season with salt and pepper.

5. Wash the vegetables and lettuce thoroughly and drain them.

6. Alternatively, dab lightly with a paper towel.

7. Cut everything into small pieces, peel the carrot well and grate with a grater.

8. Halve the avocado, remove the stone and cut the pulp into cubes.

9. Then drizzle with the juice of the lime so that there is no brown discoloration.

10. Finally cut the Gouda into cubes. Put the salad in a bowl and then add the vegetables and cheese in portions.

11. Arrange the quinoa in the middle with a dash of lime juice.

12. Now peel off the egg and place it in a free space in the bowl.
13. At the end, season everything well as you like and serve the masterpiece.

Fried Chicken Breast Pieces

Ingredients:

- Garlic Powder

- Vegetables

- Curry

- Butter

- Chicken Breast

- Salt and Pepper

Directions:

1. Cut the chicken breasts into bite-sized pieces.

2. Melt butter in a pan. Turn the heat up.

3. Add in the chicken pieces.

4. Scatter salt, pepper, garlic powder, and curry onto the chicken pieces.

5. Stir fry until the chicken becomes golden brown.

6. Remove from heat and serve. Add greens for garnishing if desired.

Ground Beef With Sliced Peppers

Ingredients:

- Onions

- Spinach

- Bell Pepper

- Coconut oil

- Ground beef

- Spices

Directions:

1. Slice onion into tiny pieces.
2. Heat coconut oil in a pan.
3. Put in the onion. Cook 'til slightly translucent.
4. Add the ground beef.
5. Put in spices of your choice.
6. Add in the spinach.

7. Stir fry until cooked to your preference.

Moroccan Meatballs

Ingredients:

Meatballs

- 2 teaspoons ground cumin

- 1 tablespoon of paprika

- ½ cup of parsley leaves (fresh and minced)

- 2 pounds of ground lamb

- ¼ cup of black pepper (ground)

- 1 teaspoon of salt

Sauce

- ½ cup parsley leaves (fresh and minced)

- 2 teaspoons ground cumin

- 2 teaspoons paprika

- 1 tablespoon coconut oil

- ¼ cup of roasted pistachios (chopped) – for garnishing

- 2 medium-sized tomatoes (diced)

- 2 cloves of garlic (crushed)

- 2 medium-sized onions (diced)

- 2/3 cup tomato paste

- 1 teaspoon salt

- 1 ½ cups of water

Directions:

1. Mix cumin, salt, pepper, parsley, and paprika in one large bowl. Stir with fork.

2. Using your hands (make sure to wash thoroughly), crumble the ground lamb into the mix until the Ingredients: are well incorporated.

3. Roll the lamb mix into balls.

4. Now, for the sauce. Heat oil in a frying pan, preferably a large one.

5. Add onion and sauté until translucent.

6. Next, add the garlic, cumin, paprika, pepper, and salt. Stir.

7. Add the tomatoes. Continue stirring.

8. Add the tomato paste, water, and parsley. Mix well until tomato paste becomes well-dissolved.

9. Let the sauce boil. After a few minutes, add the meatballs gently.

10. Cover the pan and turn the heat down slightly.

11. Cook for 40 minutes while covered. Then, remove the cover and cook for 20 more minutes.

12. Sprinkle with pistachios and serve.

Low Carb Deep Dish Pizza

Ingredients:

- 1/3 cup of heavy cream

- ¼ cup of parmesan cheese

- 3 eggs

- 4 ounces of cream cheese

- 20 slices of pepperoni

- 1 cup of shredded mozzarella

- ¼ cup of tomato sauce

- ¼ teaspoon of garlic powder

- 2 cups of shredded Italian cheese

- ½ teaspoon of oregano

- Oven should be preheated to about 375 degrees

Directions:

1. With the use of a mixing bowl, the egg and cream cheese should be beaten together till it becomes smooth

2. Stirring should then be done in parmesan, spices and heavy cream

3. 2 cups of cheese should be poured into a nonstick 13by 9 inch baking pan

4. The egg mixture will then be added on top of cheese and will be blended together so as to making the cheese get suspended in the mixture and not to get concentrated at the pan bottom

5. Baking should be done in oven for about 30 minutes

6. Remove the pan to add on layers of mozzarella and pepperoni

7. Take back to oven for another 10 minutes or till the dish turns brown

Burger Breakfast Scramble

Ingredients:

- 3 oz. of cream cheese

- 2 tablespoons of minced onions

- ½ 1b ground beef

- Salt and pepper

- 1 tablespoon of water

- 3 large eggs

Directions:

1. Brown ground beef and onions will be kept together in a skillet

2. Cream cheese will be added and will be cooked over low heat till it becomes melted

3. The eggs, water, salt and pepper will be beaten together and will be poured into a skillet

4. Scramble till it gets done

Cowboy Breakfast Skillet

Ingredients:

- Handful cilantro

- Raw cheese, optional

- Salt, to taste

- Pepper, to taste

- 1/2 lb. breakfast sausage

- 3 eggs

- 1 medium sweet potato, diced

- 1/2 avocado, diced

- Hot sauce, to taste

Directions:

1. Crank up your oven to 400ºF and allow the oven to preheat.

2. Heat an oven proof or cast iron skillet over a medium high flame and add the breakfast

sausage to it. Season with salt and pepper. Crumble it while it cooks.

3. Once the sausage is well browned, remove the crumbled sausage from the pan using a slotted spoon and set aside.

4. Add the sweet potato into the grease leftover in the pan and toss well until cooked through and crispy. Season with salt and pepper.

5. Add the cooked sausage back into the pan and mix well.

6. Using the back of a round spoon make about 3 wells in the potato and sausage mix. Take the skillet off the flame.

7. Crack an egg into a well each.

8. Place the skillet into the preheated oven and bake for about 5 minutes or until the eggs are just set.

9. Switch the oven setting to broil and cook the top off the yolks for a few minutes until the eggs are firm but still runny.

10. Carefully take the pan out of the oven and top it with some chopped cilantro and some hot sauce as per your taste.

11. Serve hot by scooping the egg, along with the sausage and greens, onto a plate. Season the egg with salt and pepper if required.

12. Enjoy!

Broccoli & Cheese Mini Egg Omelets

Ingredients:

- 1/2 teaspoon olive oil

- 2 tablespoons grated pecorino Romano

- Salt, to taste

- Freshly cracked pepper, to taste

- Cooking spray, as required

- 2 cups broccoli florets

- 1/2 cup egg whites

- 2 whole large eggs

- 2 tablespoons low fat cheddar, shredded

Directions:

1. Crank up your oven to 350 degrees F and allow the oven to preheat.

2. Pour a little water into a large vessel and place a steamer basket on it.

51

3. Add the broccoli to the basket and cover.

4. Steam for about 7 to 8 minutes or until tender.

5. Once done, crumble into smaller pieces and toss well with olive oil, pepper and salt.

6. Spray a regular cupcake tin with some cooking spray and spoon the broccoli mix into the cupcake molds.

7. Place the egg whites in a medium sized bowl.

8. Add in the whole eggs and grated pecorino Romano.

9. Whisk well to combine. Season with salt and pepper.

10. Pour the egg mix over the broccoli and fill until about 3/4ths of the mold is full.

11. Top the egg with some shredded cheddar.

12. Pop the cupcake tin into the preheated oven and bake for about 10 to 15 minutes or until cooked through.

13. Remove the cupcake tin from the oven and cool for a few minutes.

14. De-mold the mini egg omelets and serve immediately.

15. Enjoy!

Amazing And Healthy Stuffed Peppers

Ingredients:

- Black pepper

- Himalayan salt

- Paprika

- Oregano

- Dry parsley

- 250ml Fat Free Sour Cream

- 6 huge red or yellow chime peppers

- 2 medium onions

- 1.5 pounds of ground turkey

- 1 Can of diced tomatoes

- 1 container of tomato paste

Directions:

1. Preheat the broiler to 350 degrees.

2. Cut the ringer peppers in half upward and dispose of all the contents.

3. Cut onions into small pieces.

4. Mix the onions, diced tomatoes, dark pepper, Himalayan salt, paprika, oregano and the parsley in a skillet with the ground turkey and brown the meat.

5. Stuff the peppers with turkey blend (make a point to place a lot).

6. Put the peppers in the stove and prepare them for an hour.

7. Take the peppers out and present with some sharp cream on top.

Baked Chicken Balls

Ingredients:

- ¼ cup new cilantro

- Dark pepper to taste

- Salt to taste

- 5-6 medium tomatoes

- 1 huge onion

- 4lb of ground chicken

Directions:

1. Preheat the broiler for 400 Celsius.

2. Dice the tomatoes (you can purchase canned ones, however I'd avoid them, due to the preservatives).

3. Mince the onion. Throw the onions and the tomatoes in a baking dish.

4. Chop up the cilantro.

5. Put the ground chicken into a bowl.

6. Throw in and blend the cilantro, dark pepper and salt.

7. Make chicken balls about the size of your fist.

8. Put them in the baking dish and cook it for an hour

Sugar-Free Strawberry Limeade

Ingredients:

- Cold water 1 ½ cups

- Lime Juice ½ cup

- Ice cubes 6

- Strawberry extract ½ tsp

Directions:

1. Mix together the strawberry extract, lime juice, and water.

2. Add the ice cubes to a cup and pour in the strawberry mixture.

3. Sweeten with a calorie-free sweetener if desired.

Lemony Rooibos Mint Tea

Ingredients:

- Fresh mint – 5 leaves

- Sliced lemon

- Rooibos tea 6 bags

- Boiling water 1 gallon

- Sweetener 1 tbsp (do not sweeten if you just had your surgery)

Directions:

1. Bring the water to a boil. Add the tea bags and remove from the heat.
2. Pour the tea into a pitcher and stir in the remaining Ingredients:.
3. Place the pitcher in the sunlight and allow the tea to steep for at least 10 minutes.
4. Serve over ice if desired.

Low-Carb Meatloaf

Ingredients:

- 1 large egg, beaten

- 3 tablespoons taco seasoning mix

- 3 cloves garlic, minced

- 2 teaspoons ground black pepper

- 3 drops ketchup

- 2 pounds lean ground turkey

- 1 pound lean ground beef

- 1 onion, minced

- 1 carrot, shredded

- 2 cups chopped fresh spinach

Directions:

1. Preheat the oven to 375 degrees F (190 degrees C).

2. Place turkey and beef in a large bowl.

3. Add onion, carrot, spinach, egg, taco seasoning, garlic, pepper, and ketchup. Mix with your hands until blended.

4. Shape into 3 equal-sized loaves and place into a 9x13-inch baking dish.

5. Bake in the preheated oven until no longer pink in the center, about 1 1/2 hours.

6. An instant-read thermometer inserted into the center should read at least 160 degrees F (70 degrees C).

Low-Carb Meatloaf With Pork Rinds

Ingredients:

- 2 tablespoons chopped fresh parsley

- ½ teaspoon salt

- ½ teaspoon ground black pepper

- ½ teaspoon garlic powder

- 1 ½ pounds ground beef

- 1 cup crushed pork rinds

- ½ cup grated Parmesan cheese

- ⅓ cup tomato sauce

- ¼ cup chopped onion

- 1 large egg

Directions:

1. Preheat the oven to 350 degrees F (175 degrees C). Lightly grease a 9x5-inch loaf pan.

2. Combine beef, pork rinds, Parmesan cheese, tomato sauce, onion, egg, parsley, salt, pepper, and garlic powder in a bowl and shape into a loaf. Transfer to the prepared pan.

3. Bake in the preheated oven until browned and no longer pink in the center, about 1 hour.

4. An instant-read thermometer inserted into the center should read at least 160 degrees F (70 degrees C).

Gingerbread Waffles

Ingredients:

- 1/2 Tbsp baking powder

- 1 tsp ground ginger

- 1/4 cup weighty cream

- 1/4 cup water

- 1 egg

- 2 Tbsp softened spread

- 1/2 cup almond meal

- 1/2 cup vanilla whey protein powder

- 1/4 tsp salt

- 1/8 cup Splenda

Directions:

1. Heat the waffle iron.
2. In a bowl, combine as one the dry fixings.

3. Consolidate the cream and water in a glass estimating cup and afterward add the water and egg.

4. Add the dissolved spread and blend well. Add this to the dry fixings and mix to combine.

5. Pour a portion of the hitter into the waffle iron and prepare concurring to the producer's guidelines.

6. Present with whipped cream if preferred.

Hot Cinnamon Cereal

Ingredients:

- 3/4 cup wheat bran

- 1/4 cup vanilla seasoned whey protein powder

- 1 tsp cinnamon

- 1/2 cup ground flaxseeds

- 1/2 cup ground almonds

- 1/4 cup oat bran

Directions:

1. Mix the fixings together in a bowl and keep in an impenetrable container.

2. To make one serving, scoop a large portion of some the combination into a bowl and add 3/4 cup bubbling water.

3. Add a touch of salt and mix. Let sit for 2 to 3 minutes before eating.

The Swedish Keto Buns

Ingredients:

- ½ a tsp. of salt

- 1 tbsp. of baking powder

- 2 tbsp. of extra virgin olive oil

- 2 large eggs

- ½ a cup of almond flour

- 1 tbsp. of whole flax seeds

- 1 tbsp. of shelled sunflower seeds

- 2 tbsp. of Psyllium husk power

Directions:

1. Pre-heat the oven to about 400 degrees F, Mix the almond flour with the seeds, salt,

Psyllium, and baking powder inside a medium to large bowl.

2. Add the eggs, olive oil, and sour cream and mix gently for about 2 minutes.

3. Let the mix sit for about 5 minutes.

4. Cut the dough into 4 and then shape them into balls before putting them into a cake pan and make sure you use parchment papers to prevent sticking.

5. Bake the buns for about 25 minutes until they turn brown and serve when hot.

The Mini Ketogenic Donuts

Ingredients:

- 1 ½ tsp. Of coconut flour

- 1 tsp. Of baking powder

- 1 tsp. Of vanilla extract

- 4 tsp. Of erythritol extract

- 10 drops of stevia (liquid).

- 3 oz. Of cream cheese

- 3 medium to large eggs

- 3 2/3 tbsp. Of almond flour

- 1 ½ tbsp. Of coconut flour

Directions:

1. With the aid of an immersion blender, gently mix and blend all the Ingredients: thoroughly, then heat the donut maker up and spray the inside with some coconut oil.

2. Pour the batter equally into the portions of the donut maker.

3. Let the donut batter cook for about 3 minutes on one side and 3 minutes on the other side.

4. Remove the donuts from the donut maker and set the donuts aside to cool and repeat the procedure with the remaining batter if you can't finish them at once.

Cucumber Tomato Salad

Ingredients:

- 1 tablespoon lemon juice

- Salt to taste

- Ground black pepper to taste

- 2 tomatoes, chopped

- 1 cucumber, peeled and diced

- 1 onion, chopped

Directions:

1. Combine tomatoes, cucumbers, and onions in a salad bowl.

2. Season to taste with salt and black pepper.

3. Sprinkle with lemon juice. Chill.

Asparagus And Spinach Salad

Ingredients:

- 6 cups fresh spinach leaves

- 1/8 cup grated Parmesan cheese

- 1 tablespoon seasoned slivered almonds

- 1/4 cup olive oil

- 1/8 cup lemon juice

- 12 fresh asparagus spears

Directions:

1. Preheat a grill for low heat. Combine the lemon juice and olive oil on a plate.

2. Place asparagus on the plate, and roll around to coat.

3. Grill asparagus for about 5 minutes, turning at least once, and brushing with the olive oil mixture.

4. Remove from the grill, and place back onto the plate with the oil.

5. In a large bowl, combine the spinach, Parmesan cheese, and slivered almonds.

6. Cut asparagus into bite-size pieces, and add to the salad along with the lemon juice and oil from the plate. Toss to blend, then serve.

Cinnamon Coconut Peanut Butter Cookies

Ingredients:

- 1/4 cup of Butter

- 1/2 cup of Erythritol

- 2 tablespoons of Shredded Coconut

- 1 tablespoon of Cinnamon Pinch of Salt

- 1 cup of Peanut Butter

- 1 Egg

- 1/2 teaspoon of Vanilla Extract

Directions:

1. Preheat your stove to 350 degrees. Beat together your spread, peanut butter, erythritol, and egg.

2. Add your cinnamon, destroyed coconut, salt and crease everything in together.

3. Roll into balls around 1 1/2 crawls in width. Spread out on a baking sheet fixed with material paper.

4. Sprinkle with your destroyed coconut.

5. Bake roughly for 15 minutes. Edges ought to become brilliant colored.

6. Allow it to cool.

Clean Almond Butter Fat Bombs

Ingredients:

- 4 Dates

- 1/4 cup of Almond Flour

- 2 tablespoons of Mesquite Meal

- 1 cup of Almond Butter

- 1 tablespoon of Melted Unrefined Virgin

- Coconut Oil

- 1/2 teaspoon of Vanilla Extract

- 1/4 cup of Coconut Flakes

Directions:

1. Combine every one of your fixings in your food processor.

2. Roll out 1-ounce balls and put them on your material lined baking sheet.

3. Note: If your almond spread has a runny consistency, toss your consolidated fixings in

the fridge or cooler prior to folding them into individual balls.

4. Roll your balls into the garnish of your choice.

5. Store in your cooler or freezer.

Crepe Sandwich

Ingredients:

- 10g iceberg lettuce

- 4 eggs size I

- 1 tbsp honey

- Some water

- Salt and pepper

- 50g tomato

- 50g protein powder

- 20g coconut oil

- 15g ham

Directions:

1. First mix the egg white powder, eggs and honey together to form a dough.

2. Add a little water to make a nice, smooth dough. Then season the dough well.

3. Now a pan has to be heated and then add the coconut oil. It is best to spread the coconut oil with a kitchen towel.

4. Now set the heat level to medium heat and then add a little thin dough to the pan.

5. Give the dough enough time to bake well.

6. Turn after 2 minutes and bake the other side.

7. After another 2 minutes, remove from the pan and place on a plate with a kitchen towel on it to cool.

8. Wash the tomatoes and lettuce with hot water and cut them into pieces.

9. Also cut the ham into small pieces. The crepe can now be topped and then consumed.

10. If you prefer it warm, you can warm up the finished sandwiches in a pan beforehand.

Protein Pancakes

Ingredients:

- 5g desiccated coconut

- 1 egg size L

- 1 teaspoon vanilla extract

- 1 teaspoon cocoa powder (raw)

- 1 teaspoon baking powder

- 90ml coconut milk

- 50g cream cheese

- 30g protein powder (best: chocolate)

- 15ml coconut oil

Directions:

1. Mix the coke milk with the cream cheese, egg, vanilla extract, protein and baking powder in a large bowl.

2. The whole thing has to be stirred until a thick chocolate mass is formed.

3. After the dough has the right consistency, heat a pan and add the coconut oil, spread it with a kitchen towel and let it melt.

4. Then lower it to the medium level, otherwise the pancakes will burn too quickly.

5. Divide the dough evenly and put a small ladle with dough in each pan.

6. Now fry the pancake until it has a light golden brown color. Then turn it over and do the same with the other side.

7. Take the finished pancakes out of the pan and drain on a kitchen towel.

8. As soon as 5 pancakes are stacked on top of each other, this stack can be garnished as desired.

9. Various fruits or a sugar-free chocolate icing are suitable for this. Finally, sprinkle with desiccated coconut.

Primal Chili Cheese Dogs

Ingredients:

- 15 ounces roasted tomatoes

- 1 teaspoon chili powder

- 2 cloves of garlic (minced)

- 2 Chipotle Peppers (drained and sliced)

- 3 ounces of cheddar cheese (raw and sharp, grated)

- ½ teaspoon cocoa powder (optional)

- 6 Hotdogs (preferably sugar-free)

- Cooking oil of your choice

- 1 pound of ground beef

- 3 sweet potatoes (sliced in half, lengthwise)

- Salt and pepper

- ½ onion (red, diced)

Directions:

1. Preheat the oven to 450 degrees F.

2. Coat the sweet potatoes with cooking oil.

3. Put them in baking sheets and roast inside the ovens 'til skins are a bit charred and the insides become soft.

4. While sweet potatoes are baking, begin cooking the chili.

5. Heat oil in a pan. Add the garlic and onions. Sauté for about 10 minutes.

6. Add the Chipotle peppers, then the tomatoes, cocoa powder, chili powder, salt, and pepper.

7. Put the ground beef into the pan. Break up any big chunks with a spatula. Cook until the beef is well done.

8. After the sweet potatoes are done, remove them from the baking sheet and use the same sheets for roasting the hotdogs.

9. Roast them in the oven for about 7 minutes.

10. While roasting the dogs, prepare the potatoes by scooping out the insides (save them for another recipe).

11. Assembly: place the hotdog on top of the prepared potato skin.

12. Put in the chili and use cheese as topping.

Enchilada Chicken Mango Salad

Ingredients:

- ½ avocado (diced)

- 1 small piece of hearts of romaine (shredded)

- Salt and pepper

- 1 large mango (peeled, diced)

- 1-2 cups of enchilada chicken (you can use leftovers)

Directions:

1. Chop the romaine.
2. Put the chicken on top of it.
3. Top with mango and avocado.
4. Sprinkle with a bit of salt and pepper.

Spinach Salad With Hot Bacon Dressing

Ingredients:

- 2 hardboiled eggs, chopped

- 4 slices of bacon

- ¼ c chopped onion

- 1 bag of fresh baby spinach

- Salt and pepper

- 1 Pkg. Splenda

- ¼ cup of vinegar

Directions:

1. Bacon will be cooked and will be allowed to drain on a paper, bacon grease should then be greased in a pan

2. Vinegar, pepper and splenda to bacon grease will be added

3. Stirring and heating will be done slowly till it boils

4. Spinach should then be teared into salad sized pieces and tossed with egg, crumbled bacon and onion

5. Pour on hot dressing immediately and then toss lightly

Drunken Chicken

Ingredients:

- 1 Tablespoon Brown Sugar Twin

- 1 tablespoon of parsley

- 1 clove garlic, crushed

- ½ small onion, minced

- 1 tablespoon of butter

- 4 boneless and skinless chicken breasts

- 4 tablespoons of Gin

- ¼ cup of red wine

- ½ cup of chicken stock

- 1 tablespoon of mustard

Directions:

1. Oven should be preheated to about 350 degrees

2. With the use of a large skillet, chicken and butter will be sauté till the chicken becomes brownish

3. Get the chicken removed and set it aside

4. Onion should then be added to the skillet, sauté up till it becomes soft

5. The remaining Ingredients: will be puree in a blender, add up to skillet and heat through

6. Chicken should then be placed in a baking dish, pour the mixture on top

7. Baking should be done 15 to 20 minutes for boneless breast and 30 to 40 minutes for bone in split breasts

Tex-Mex Scramble

Ingredients:

- 1/8 cup chopped red onion

- 1/4 cup frozen spinach, thawed and drained

- 1 cherry tomato, diced

- 3 jalapeno pepper slices, chopped

- 1 tablespoon salsa

- 1 tablespoon oil of your choice

- 1/2 slice cheddar

- 3 eggs

- 1/8 cup chopped green pepper

- 1 tablespoon water

Directions:

1. Heat a cast iron skillet over a medium flame. Add in the oil and heat until lightly smoking.

2. Combine the eggs, pepper, tomatoes, jalapenos, water, onion and spinach together in a medium mixing bowl and whisk well until well combined.
3. Pour the mix onto the hot pan and cook until the eggs reach the consistency you like, stirring to scramble the egg.
4. When the eggs are just done, turn the flame off and place the cheddar cheese slice on the eggs.
5. Cover the skillet with a lid and let it sit for about 5 minutes.
6. Serve immediately, topped with a tablespoon of salsa.
7. Enjoy!

Savory Cheese Chive Waffles

Ingredients:

- ½ tablespoon chives

- ½ teaspoon onion powder

- ½ teaspoon garlic powder

- ¼ teaspoon pepper

- 1/2 cup raw cauliflower, processed into a fine crumb

- 1/6 cup Parmesan cheese, shredded

- 1/2 cup processed mozzarella shredded cheese

- 1 egg

Directions:

1. Prepare the waffle batter by combining all the Ingredients: together in a large mixing bowl. Whisk until it forms a uniformly thick batter.

2. Heat a waffle maker until heated through.

3. Pour about 1/4th of the prepared batter on the girdle. Shut the waffle maker and set the time for about 6 minutes.

4. After the fourth minute, lightly peak at the waffles cooking. If the waffle sticks, cook it for a little longer.

5. Once cooked, slowly extract the waffle from the waffle maker and cool it on the plate.

6. Serve immediately with a side of eggs cooked sunny side up.

7. Enjoy!

Garlic Mashed Cauliflower

Ingredients:

- 1cup new parsley

- Salt and pepper (to taste)

- 500g of new cauliflower 1 medium head

- 2 cloves of new garlic

Directions:

1. Steam the cauliflower until it is delicate. It ought to be not difficult to penetrate it with a fork.

2. Crush the garlic utilizing garlic press.

3. Mash the cauliflower.

4. Mix in the garlic, parsley and spices.

5. Enjoy!

Chicken Spaghetti Squash

Ingredients:

- 1 cup finely cleaved new tomatoes

- 1 tbsp. dried basil

- ½ cup new parsley

- 1 tbsp. dried oregano

- 1lb additional lean ground chicken

- Salt and pepper to taste

- 1 tsp Coconut Oil

- 1 cup slashed onion

- 5 cloves minced garlic

- 1 cup cut mushrooms

Directions:

1. Put the ground chicken in a bowl and blend in 1 tsp. of salt, 1 tbsp. of dark pepper and 1 tbsp. of garlic powder.

2. Put a skillet on medium and shower some Pam.

3. Sautee mushrooms, garlic and onion in the pan.

4. When the onions are straightforward add the tomatoes, parsley, oregano and basil.

5. Set the hotness on low and add 1/4 cup of water.

6. Allow the sauce to stew, while mixing occasionally.

7. In another container, brown the chicken on medium hotness. Channel any fat.

8. When the meat is done, add it to the sauce and mix all that together.

9. Serve on top of spaghetti squash.

Coco-Orange Cocktail

Ingredients:

- Natural sweetening syrup 2 tbs (optional)

- Lime juice 5 tbs

- Rock salt dash

- Wedge of lemon

- Squeezed orange juice 2 tbs

- Coconut water 4 tbs

Directions:

1. Add the orange juice, coconut water, syrup and lime juice to a shaker and shake vigorously for about 20 seconds.

2. Pour the drink over some ice.

3. Sprinkle a dash of salt and serve with a lemon wedge if desired

Grandma's Chicken Soup

Ingredients:

- Bay leaf 2

- Garlic cloves 5

- Celery stalks 2

- Peeled carrots 2

- Quartered onion 1

- Whole chicken 1

- Water to fill cover Ingredients:

- Lemon 2 slices

- Apple cider vinegar 1 tbs

- Peppercorns ½ tsp

- Sea salt 2 tsp

- Parsley 5 stems

- Thyme 4 sprigs

Directions:

1. Place a six eight-quart pot with a tight lid on a stovetop. Clean the chicken thoroughly and remove any visible fat.

2. Add all the Ingredients: to your pot and add enough water into it to cover everything. Cover the pot and allow the liquid to come to a boil.

3. Reduce the heat and let it simmer for four hours while you carry on with your daily activities. The pot should stay covered so that the liquid doesn't evaporate.

4. Remember to remove chicken after two hours so that it doesn't overcook and add the bones back into the pot.

5. You can save the meat for other uses.

6. Strain the liquid through a colander and discard any solids.

7. Allow the stock to come to room temperature and then store it in quart containers in the fridge for three days.

Bacon Egg With Cheese Muffins

Ingredients:

- ½ a tsp. of salt

- ½ a cup of water

- 5 beaten eggs

- 3 stripped bacon

- ½ a cup of shredded cheddar cheese

- 1 cup of cottage cheese

- ¾ cup of grated Parmesan cheese

- ¼ of a cup of coconut flour

- 2/3 of a cup of almond flour

- 1 tbsp. of baking powder

Directions:

1. Pre-heat your oven to about 400 degrees F, and grease your muffin cups.

2. Get a mixing bowl and inside mix the cottage cheese, with Parmesan cheese, almond flour,

coconut flour, salt, water, baking powder, and the egg that has just been beaten.

3. Mix the crumbled bacon alongside the cheddar cheese. Fill up the muffin cups until they are half or ¾ full, then sprinkle the muffin tops with extra cheddar cheese (shredded) this is optional.

4. Bake for about 30 minutes, until the muffins have become light brown and serve them hot or cold for few minutes at room temperature before serving.

The Delicious Ketogenic Cheese And Bacon Rolls

Ingredients:

- 1 ½ tsp. of baking powder

- ½ a cup of 3 large eggs mozzarella grated cheese

- ½ tsp. of salt

- ½ tsp. of red pepper

- 5 oz. of Bacon (must be diced into 6)

- 2 tsp. of sesame seeds

- 1 cup of grated cheddar cheese

- 1 tbsp. of Psyllium seeds

- 2 tbsp. of cream cheese

Directions:

1. Pre-heat your oven to about 355 degrees F, and inside a non-sticky frying pan, sauté the diced bacon over medium to high heat, and

until the bacon starts to brown turn off the heat at this point.

2. Add your cream cheese inside the bacon, and allow the cheese to become soften while the bacon is cooling.

3. Place the cream cheese alongside the bacon inside a food processor, and add the remainder of the Ingredients: (keep a spoonful of the bacon aside as top up for the rolls).

4. Then, blend the mix in the processor at medium speed for around 5 minutes, until the Ingredients: become well combined.

5. Next, spoon the blended mix into 12 equal piles, on a lined baking dish, before you sprinkle the remaining bacon on top of every roll.

6. Bake the rolls for about 16 minutes, until they become puffed up and golden in color.

7. You can store them while hot or keep them in the refrigerator.

Artichoke Soup

Ingredients:

- 1.5 cups heavy whipping cream

- 4 tbsp cream cheese with spinach and artichoke

- 2 cups cheddar cheese, shredded

- 1 tbsp celery, diced

- 1 tsp olive oil

- 1 cup chicken broth

Directions:

1. Saute celery in olive oil until tender. Add chicken broth and simmer 5 minutes.

2. Whisk in heavy cream and cream cheese until smooth. Simmer 5 minutes, or until it starts to thicken.

3. Gradually whisk in cheddar cheese until smooth. Season with salt and pepper.

Tomato Soup

Ingredients:

- 1 cup heavy cream

- Salt and pepper, to taste

- 2 tablespoons parsley, minced, optional

- 2 tablespoons butter

- 1/2 cup onion, 2 3/4 ounces

- 28 ounce can diced tomatoes, undrained

- 2 cups chicken broth

Directions:

1. In a 3-quart pot, sauté the onion in butter until tender.
2. Add the tomatoes, with their liquid, and broth; bring to a boil.

3. Simmer 5 minutes. Puree with a stick blender until smooth.
4. Stir in the cream and adjust the seasoning. Stir in the parsley and serve.

Coconut Blackberry Fat Bombs

Ingredients:

- 1 cup of Coconut Oil

- 1/2 teaspoon of Sweet Leaf Stevia Drops

- 1/2 cup of Fresh or Frozen Blackberries

- 1 cup of Coconut Butter

- 1 tablespoon of Lemon Juice

- 1/4 teaspoon of Vanilla Powder or 1/2 teaspoon of Vanilla Extract

Directions:

1. Place your coconut margarine, coconut oil, and blackberries (whenever frozen) in a pot and hotness over a medium hotness until well combined.

2. In your food processor or little blender, add your coconut oil blend and remaining fixings. Process until smooth. Division might happen

on the off chance that coconut oil blend is excessively hot. In the case of utilizing new berries, there is no compelling reason to cook them with the coconut oil and butter.

3. Spread out into a little measured dish fixed with material paper (I utilized a 6x6-inch container)

4. Refrigerate for one hour or until your blend has hardened.

5. Remove from your compartment and cut into squares.

6. Store shrouded in your refrigerator.

Coconut Macaroons

Ingredients:

- 1 teaspoon of Vanilla

- 2 cups of Unsweetened Coconut

- 1/2 teaspoon of EZ-Sweet

- 4 Egg Whites

- 4 1/2 teaspoons of Water

Directions:

1. Combine your egg whites and liquids.

2. Add your coconut and blend together.

3. Spread on your lubed pie pan.

4. Preheat your broiler to 375 degrees

5. Whenever you put in your macaroons lessen hotness to 325 degrees and prepare for roughly 14 minutes.

Protein Waffles

Ingredients:

- 5g maple syrup

- 2 eggs size m

- Some water

- 50ml milk (1.5% fat)

- 30g protein powder (vanilla)

- 10g quark

- 5g honey

Directions:

1. Heat the waffle iron and brush with a little coconut oil.

2. Then put the quark, milk, protein powder, eggs, honey and water in a bowl and mix well until you get a smooth dough.

3. Then pour the batter into the waffle iron in portions (about 1 ladle and distribute it

thoroughly). Bake the waffle until it is golden brown.

4. Then divide the whole dough evenly and bake the waffles, let them cool, shape into a stack and garnish with maple syrup.

Cheese Omelet

Ingredients:

- 1 clove of garlic

- 1 onion (small)

- 1 package of paprika curd cheese

- Nutmeg (grated)

- Salt and pepper

- 250g young leaf spinach

- 60g parmesan cheese

- 8 eggs size m

- 3 tbsp oil

Directions:

1. Wash the spinach and dry it well. Heat 1 tablespoon of oil in a saucepan and then add the onions and garlic and let simmer for 2 minutes. Add the spinach, collapse in the pan

and season to taste. After seasoning, put the spinach in a colander and drain.

2. Grate the parmesan. Separate the eggs, beat the egg whites until stiff. Fold the egg yolks with 50g Parmesan into the egg white mixture and then add the spinach. Season the mixture properly. Heat an ovenproof pan and then add the oil. At the same time, preheat the oven to 180 ° C fan-assisted air.

3. Pour the egg white mixture into the pan and let it set on medium heat for about 3 minutes.

4. Spread the rest of the cheese generously on the omelets and place everything in the preheated oven.

5. Let it stand there for about 10 minutes.

6. Season the quark to taste and serve together when the omelet is finished.

Coconut And Almond Bread

Ingredients:

- 1 ½ teaspoons baking soda

- ¼ cup of coconut oil

- 5 eggs

- 1 tablespoon apple cider vinegar

- 1 tablespoon honey

- 1 ½ cups of almond flour

- 2 tablespoons of coconut flour

- ¼ teaspoon salt

- ¼ cup flaxseed meal

Directions:

1. Preheat the oven to 350 degrees F.
2. Grease the loaf pan you'll use.

3. Put in the almond flour, flaxseed meal, baking soda, coconut flour, and salt in the food processor.

4. Pulse the mixture.

5. Add the eggs, honey, oil, and vinegar. Pulse it again.

6. Transfer the resulting batter into the greased oil pan. Then, bake for about 30 minutes.

Topside Rolls

Ingredients:

- 1/8 teaspoon cream of tartar

- 3 ounces of cream cheese (full-fat, cold and cubed)

- 1/8 teaspoon salt

- Cooking Spray

- 3 large eggs

Directions:

1. Preheat the oven to 350 degrees F.

2. Use parchment to line a cookie sheet. Spray lightly with cooking spray.

3. Separate the egg yolks from the whites.

4. Whip the egg whites with the cream of tartar.

5. Whip the yolks, salt, and cream cheese.

6. Mix the egg white mixture with the egg yolk mixture batch by batch. Place a mound of the

former on top of the latter. Then, fold the latter over the mound.

7. Spoon large mounds of the resulting mixture and put them into the prepared baking sheets. Use a spatula to lightly flatten each mound.

8. Bake for about 30-40 minutes.

Low Carbs Cauliflower Hash Brown

Ingredients:

- 3 oz. chopped onion

- 4 slices of bacon, chopped

- Salt and pepper

- 1 tablespoon, soften

Directions:

1. Bacon and onion should be sauté in a skillet till it becomes brownish

2. Cauliflower should then be added and stirring will be done till it becomes brown and tender all over

3. Add butter through the cooking

4. Seasoning will be done to taste using salt and pepper

Swedish Breakfast Buns

Ingredients:

- ¼ teaspoon salt

- ½ teaspoon baking powder

- 1 tablespoon olive oil

- ¼ cup sour cream

- 1 eggs

- 6 tablespoons almond flour

- ½ tablespoon sunflower seeds, shells removed

- ½ tablespoon whole flax seeds

- 1 tablespoon psyllium husk powder

Directions:

1. Crank up your oven to 400°F and allow the oven to preheat.

2. Combine the almond flour, psyllium husk, baking powder, sunflower seeds, flax seeds and salt together in a bowl.

3. In a small mixing bowl whisk together the egg, sour cream and olive oil.

4. Once combined, pour the wet Ingredients: into the dry Ingredients: and mix well to form a soft dough.

5. Cover and set aside for about 5 minutes.

6. Divide the dough into 4 equal parts and shape into smooth rounds.

7. Place the dough balls in a cake pan (a 9 inch circular cake pan should do).

8. Pop the cake pan into the preheated oven and bake for about 20 to 25 minutes, or until they are well browned.

9. Cool and serve with eggs cooked to your preference.

10. Enjoy!

Eggs Benedict With A Lazy Hollandaise Sauce

Ingredients:

- 2 tablespoons butter

- 1 recipe Lazy Hollandaise Sauce (mentioned below)

- 1 egg

- 1 slice of ham

Directions:

1. Heat a small pan over a medium flame. Add in the butter and when well heated through, add in the egg and scramble the egg inn it. Do not scramble it too much and ensure that the egg cooks in single mass.

2. Flip the eggs over to cook the other side through. Fold once (or more than once) to create a small muffin like structure with the egg. Cool for about 3 minutes.

3. Cut the ham into a circle that will fit the diameter of the "egg muffin".
4. Place the egg muffin on the slice of ham and serve immediately topped with some hollandaise.
5. Enjoy!

Baked Sweet French Fries

Ingredients:

- 2-3 enormous sweet potatoes

- 1 tsp. Coconut oil

- 1 tsp. Ground garlic

- 1 tsp. Ground chili

- Salt (to taste)

Directions:

1. Cut the potatoes into a French fry shape.
2. Lightly splash them with Pam and mix.
3. Add the flavors and blend again.
4. Place the fries on a baking dish in one layer.
5. Bake for 1 hour on 375.
6. You can serve this formula with our Dill Garlic Dip (pg. 116).

Vitamin C Infused Tropical Delight

Ingredients:

- Limes 2

- Lemon 1

- Grapefruits 5

- Handful of ginger

- Pineapple ¼

Directions:

1. Remove the tops and bottoms from the grapefruits. Cut around the edges of the peeling.

2. Make sure you don't cut away the pith. This holds a lot of nutrients.

3. Do the same thing with the lemon, limes, and pineapple.

4. Juice the grapefruits, ginger, limes, and lemon. Lastly, juice the pineapple.

5. Mix well with the remaining the ginger and serve over ice. Enjoy.

Chico-Banana Protein Shake

Ingredients:

- Chocolate whey isolate protein powder ¼ cup

- PB2 powder ¼ cup

- Light soy milk 1 cup

- Ice cubes – 5 cubes

- Frozen sliced banana 1

Directions:

1. Place all of the Ingredients: in a high-speed blender and mix until everything is smooth and creamy.

Low-Carb Beef And Turkey Meatloaf

Ingredients:

- 1 tablespoon chili powder

- 1 tablespoon garlic powder

- 1 tablespoon onion powder

- 1 teaspoon salt, or to taste

- 1 teaspoon ground black pepper, or to taste

- 1 ½ pounds lean ground beef

- 1 pound ground turkey

- 3 large eggs

- 1 cup shredded sharp Cheddar cheese

- 2 tablespoons Worcestershire sauce

- 2 tablespoons Italian seasoning

Directions:

1. Preheat the oven to 350 degrees F (175 degrees C). Spray a loaf dish with cooking spray.

2. Mix ground beef, ground turkey, eggs, Cheddar cheese, Worcestershire, Italian seasoning, chili powder, garlic powder, onion powder, salt, and pepper thoroughly in a large mixing bowl. Place in the prepared pan. Cover.

3. Bake in the preheated oven until no longer pink in the center, about 1 hour.

4. An instant-read thermometer inserted into the center should read at least 160 degrees F (70 degrees C).

Low-Carb Fauxtato Salad

Ingredients:

- 2 tablespoons dill pickle relish

- 2 tablespoons diced green onion

- 1 tablespoon prepared yellow mustard

- salt and ground black pepper to taste

- 1 head cauliflower, cut into bite-size pieces

- 4 hard-boiled eggs, chopped

- ½ cup mayonnaise, or more to taste

Directions:

1. Place a steamer insert into a saucepan and fill with water to just below the bottom of the steamer. Bring water to a boil.

2. Add cauliflower, cover, and steam until tender, about 5 minutes.

3. Mix cauliflower, eggs, mayonnaise, dill pickle relish, green onion, mustard, salt, and pepper together in a bowl.

Broccoli And Onion Soup

Ingredients:

- 2 cups of fresh broccoli florets

- 5 cups of water

- 1 cup of whipping cream

- 1 large tbsp chicken soup powder

- 1 large red onion

- 2 tbsp coconut oil

- 1 tbsp tamari sauce

Directions:

1. Start with a saute of the red onions in coconut oil.

2. Then add the water and broccoli. Cook for 10-12 minutes.

3. Puree the soup with a immersion blender.

4. Add the whipping cream at the end and only on low heat. Serve hot.

Spinach Soup

Ingredients:

- 1/2 teaspoon salt

- 1/4 teaspoon pepper

- 2 1/2 cups vegetable broth

- 2 ounces fresh baby spinach, roughly chopped, about 4 cups loosely packed

- 1/2 cup heavy cream, room temperature

- 1 tablespoon butter

- 6 ounces fresh mushrooms, sliced

- 1 tablespoon onion, minced

- 1 clove garlic, minced

Directions:

1. Sauté the mushrooms, onion, garlic and seasonings in butter in a large saucepan until lightly browned, 5 minutes.

2. Add the broth and wine; cook on high heat
    until reduced by half, about 4 minutes.
    Remove from the heat and put half of the
    soup in a small, deep bowl.
3. Puree the soup in the bowl with a blender.
    Return the puree to the pot and heat until the
    soup is hot.
4. Stir in the spinach and cream; heat through
    for a minute and serve.

Coconut Raspberry Slice

Ingredients:

Biscuit layer:

- 1 Large Egg

- 2 cups of Almond Meal

- 1 tablespoon of Butter (Room Temperature)

- 1/2 teaspoon of Baking Soda

Coconut layer:

- 1 cup of Unsweetened Coconut Milk (Canned)
  1/3 cup of Powdered Erythritol

- 1/4 cup of Coconut Oil

- 1 teaspoon of Vanilla Bean Powder

- 3 cups of Unsweetened Desiccated Coconut

- Pinch of Sea Salt

Raspberry layer:

- 1 teaspoon of Powdered Erythritol

- 2 tablespoons of Water

- 1 cup of Raspberries

- 3 tablespoons of Chia Seeds

Chocolate layer:

- 4 ounces of 85% Dark Chocolate

Directions:

1. Preheat your stove to 350 degrees. Join all your roll layer fixings in a bowl and blend until your batter structures.

2. Line a 8×8 inch baking dish or brownie container with your material paper. Equally press your bread roll mixture into the dish to shape the base. Heat in the stove for roughly 15 minutes, until softly sautéed and cooked through. Permit it to cool.

3. Make your raspberry layer by adding each of your fixings into a little estimated dish and mix over a low hotness. Separate your

raspberries as they cook so a jam structures. Continue to mix for around 5 minutes, until thickened. Permit it to cool.

4. On a medium hotness blend your coconut milk and coconut oil until combined.

   5. Mix every one of your excess elements for the coconut layer together. Add your coconut milk and oil combination to the dry fixings and join well.

5. Add your coconut blend to your cooled bread roll base and spread equitably. Place in your cooler until set (around 60 minutes). When the coconut layer is hard, spread the raspberry layer over its highest point and return to the cooler to set (around 1 hour).

6. Break your chocolate bar into little measured pieces, then, at that point, place in a reasonable bowl and dissolve in your microwave (roughly 3 minutes). Pour your

chocolate onto the raspberry layer and return to the cooler to set.

7. Remove from your cooler around 30 minutes prior to serving. The cuts can be put away in the fridge for around a week or in the cooler for around 3 months.

Coconut Strawberry-Filled Fat Bombs

Ingredients:

- 1 tablespoons of Unsweetened Shredded Coconut

- 1/2 tablespoon of Cocoa Powder

- 1/3 cup of Coconut Oil + 1 tablespoon
  8 to 10 drops of Liquid Stevia

- 1/3 cup of Coconut Butter

- 1/3 cup of Diced Fresh Strawberries

Directions:

1. In your bain-marie, add your coconut margarine, 1/3 cup of coconut oil, cocoa powder, and a couple of drops of fluid stevia. Heat until completely melted.

2. Meanwhile, in your little estimated griddle, add your new strawberries and a couple of spoonfuls of water.

3. Cook over a medium hotness until delicate. Crush with a fork.

4. Add the berries to a blender with 1 tablespoon of dissolved coconut oil and a couple of more drops of fluid stevia. Mix until smooth.

5. Fill your molds with the liquefied coconut combination.

6. Add around 1 teaspoon of the strawberry combination into each form.

7. Sprinkle with a couple of smidgens of unsweetened coconut.

8. Place in your cooler until completely solidified; no less than several hours or short-term.

9. Jump out of the molds and store in an impenetrable compartment in the refrigerator.

Mushroom Omelet

Ingredients:

- 5g parsley

- 1 tbsp olive oil

- 1 spring onion

- Sea salt and pepper

- 70g mushrooms

- 50ml cream

- 40g onion

- 8 eggs size m

Directions:

1. First, put the eggs in a bowl. Then whisk together with the cream.

2. Peel the onion and cut into rings.

3. At the same time, thoroughly clean the mushrooms and spring onions and cut them into slices.

4. Wash the parsley, shake dry and chop finely.

5. Heat a pan and then add oil. Fry the onion with the mushrooms in it.

6. After both are golden brown, remove and set aside.

7. Now season the eggs, put half of them in the pan and fry them.

8. The heat should be on the medium level, otherwise the underside will burn too easily.

9. Now place the spring onion, the parsley and the fried onions with the mushrooms on the egg mixture and cover with the remaining egg.

10. Then the omelet has to falter first. As soon as the omelet is sufficiently thick, take the omelet out of the pan and consume.

Quinoa With Egg And Avocado

Ingredients:

- 2 eggs size m

- 1 lime

- Sea salt and pepper

- 120g avocado

- 50g quinoa

- 10g chia seeds

Directions:

1. Rinse the avocado, cut in half and remove from the skin. Cut the pulp into approx. 1cm thick strips.

2. Bring water to a boil in a saucepan and boil the eggs hard for 10 minutes. Then quench and remove the peel. Cut the eggs into approx. 1cm thick slices.

3. Then rinse the quinoa thoroughly under running water in a sieve, place in a saucepan and cover with water. Cook for 10 minutes until al dente and then drain through a sieve.

4. Wash the lime off with hot water, rub some peel and then drizzle the quinoa with the juice. Season to taste with sea salt and pepper.

5. Place the avocado and eggs on top of the quinoa and sprinkle with the chia seeds. Season to taste with the grated lime zest, a few splashes of lime juice, sea salt and pepper.